EMERGENCY EVACUATION

BARBARA SALSBURY

Deseret Book Company
Salt Lake City, Utah

First printing April 1986

Library of Congress Cataloging-in-Publication Data

Salsbury, Barbara, 1937-
    Emergency evacuation.
    1. Evacuation of civilians.   2. Survival skills.
3. Disaster relief.   I. Title.
UA 926.5.S35   1986   363.348   86-6399
    ISBN 0-87579-037-2 (pbk.)

Printed in the United States of America   93163-6491

10   9   8   7   6   5   4   3   2   1

CONTENTS

Foreword		v
1 Preparing for an Evacuation		1
Analyze the Risks	3	
Locate Your Evacuation Shelter	4	
Lag Time	5	
2 The Seventy-Two-Hour Evacuation Kit		7
The Container	7	
Keep Your Kits Accessible	9	
Label Your Kits	10	
Maintain Your Kits	10	
3 Food		12
Foods Suitable for Evacuation Kits	13	
A Seventy-Two-Hour Menu	15	
Foods Not Suitable for Evacuation Kits	15	
Food for a Baby or Toddler	16	
Containers, Utensils, and Equipment	17	
Planning Your Kit	18	
Practice Sessions	18	
4 Water		20
Water Containers	20	
Purifying Water	21	
5 Shelter, Clothing, Heat, and Light		23
Shelter	23	
Blankets	23	
Heat	25	
Light	25	
Clothing	26	
Clothes for a Baby or Toddler	27	

6 Sanitation and First Aid   29
      Personal Hygiene   30
      First Aid   30
7 Miscellaneous Items   32
      Important Documents   32
      Money   33
      Morale Boosters   34
      Important Phone Numbers   34
      The Don't-Forget List   35
      Other Items   35
8 Communications   36
9 Neighborhood Cooperation   38
      The Care-in-a-Crisis Program   38
10 Evacuation   40
      Transportation   40
      What If You Have to Walk Out?   41
      Practice Sessions   41
      Pets   41
      Leaving Your Home   42
      Returning Home   42
    Forms
      Neighborhood Evaluation   44
      Worksheet for 72-Hour Evacuation Kit   46
      Food and Equipment to Be Purchased   48
      Care-in-a-Crisis Plan   56
      Family Information   58

FOREWORD

Now and then we are given various steps in emergency preparedness by those in the know, and between the covers of this book are some excellent guidelines and ideas written in a fresh new style by Barbara Salsbury. She points out the steps that families and individuals can take to provide them with the knowledge and security needed in time of stress. Preparedness on the family level is of much value to the local and state emergency management.

A. Deon Harris
Director of Emergency Services,
  Bannock County, Idaho
Graduate of National Emergency
  Training Center
President of Region 10, United States
  Civil Defense Council

CHAPTER ONE

PREPARING FOR AN EVACUATION

Civil Defense. Disaster. Crisis. Emergency. These words may give you feelings of apathy or terror, depending on whether or not you have experienced the things the words describe. Most disasters are sudden and unexpected, and people are seldom prepared for the problems a disaster may bring. Reporter Clarence Peterson summed up the attitude most people have as he wrote about one disaster: "The victims had been exposed to countless disasters. They had read newspaper accounts of train wrecks, plane crashes, hotel fires, and hurricanes, and seen them on television, just as we would now read and gape at pictures of what happened to them. It is safe to say that many of them had also seen 'The Poseidon Adventure,' 'The Towering Inferno,' or any of a dozen disaster films, but for all that, disasters are what happen to somebody else.

"We say, 'My hair is a disaster!' or 'The kids' room is a disaster!' or 'The vacation was an *absolute* disaster!'—expressions that devalue the currency of disaster, reducing it to small change that fits snugly into a pocket of the mind not far from those in which fear and foreboding reside." (*Chicago Tribune*, May 26, 1982.)

Unfortunately, what we learn from disaster movies and even news reports may have little meaning for us personally. Most of us cling to the hope that if we don't think about disaster, it will never happen to us. Disaster is what happens only to somebody else.

But the fact is, sooner or later you may be forced to leave your home, even if only temporarily, because of some kind of emergency. The world we live in is dangerous. Earthquakes, tornadoes, fires, floods, and hurricanes can occur almost anywhere and at any time. And to the natural disasters, we can add a long list of man-made problems, such as explosions, leakage of hazardous chemicals or radioactive waste, and the atomic bomb.

A few recent disasters are still fresh in memory. Who can forget the deadly chemical leaks in India; the train carrying toxic chemicals that exploded in Louisiana, forcing an entire community to evacuate; the Three-Mile Island incident? Recently a small town in Texas was evacuated because of life-threatening fires in oil-storage tanks. After the danger was over, one reporter noted: "The citizens wearily returned to their homes knowing it can—and probably will—happen again."

It is difficult to understand how people can be apathetic about preparing for disaster. The Congressional Research Service Report released in March 1985 reports that in 1982 there were 11,368 chemical manufacturing plants in the United States, most of them in the nation's 335 metropolitan areas, where 75.8 percent of the population lived in 1980. We may conclude that three of every four people live near a chemical plant. We don't know which plants are potentially dangerous. But some certainly are.

When disaster strikes, invariably people are forced to flee from their homes. Perhaps you will never have to do this. But disasters are increasing, not decreasing, throughout the world. Shouldn't you be prepared so that if you have to leave your home, even if only for a few hours, you can do so with a minimum of discomfort? The fact is, your preparation may even save your life or the lives of your family.

But in case of a disaster, won't the government come to the rescue? The sad truth is that Civil Defense, with benefits and programs for the individual, for the most part is dead. There are still a few fallout shelters from the 1950s scattered around the country, but not many people pay any attention to them anymore, let alone maintain them. The yellow-and-black shelter signs look out in sad silence from their useless vigil on posts and buildings. They are insignias of security no longer. Most emergency food rations and medical supplies in these shelters have long ago disappeared.

State and city governments may have people whose job it is to take care of emergencies, but they are trained to deal with crowds, not individuals. And if you think that the Red Cross or Salvation Army will come running to the rescue, think again. Such agencies do help, but they have to rely largely on volunteer labor. In a disaster, that may mean bringing in people from outside the disaster area. And that takes time. What will you do until help arrives?

There are choices you can make when faced with disasters. You can put on a long, sad face and resign yourself to doom, or you can take the attitude that despite the problems, there are positive actions you can take. Practical preparation could very well make the difference between surviving and coping, or chaos!

The emphasis of this manual is *not* "survivalism" or preparation for doomsday! It is not based on the theory that the world is falling apart; that you need an arms stockpile; or that you need to be taught wilderness survival so you can flee to the hills for safety. Home storage, emergency preparedness, and seventy-two-hour evacuations all have *different* parameters, guidelines, and rules to follow. *Emergency Evacuation* offers practical solutions to meet individual needs if you are forced to evacuate your home for any reason.

Analyze the Risks

Analyze the risks in your area. A crisis needs to happen only once! When it does, it's too late to start making lists and gathering equipment that would have insured your survival. *Now* is the time to prepare!

Assess your neighborhood so that you can plan—not panic. As you become aware of the problems that could occur in your neighborhood, the chance that you could be forced to evacuate your home will be brought sharply into focus in your mind. When you combine these problems with the possibility of natural disasters, your understanding of the need to prepare an individual evacuation plan and kit becomes even more pronounced. This is not a fanatical concept, but the positive attitude of having the foresight to assess a potential problem and deal with it! Determine the proximity of freeways, railroads, and factories to your home. As you note these, think of the specific problems they could cause. For example, are you aware that toxic materials are often transported by truck? If a spill or leak occurs on a nearby highway, you could be evacuated. Railroads also carry substances that could be threatening. Take time to fill out the Neighborhood Evaluation worksheet on page 44 as you draw up your plan. Once it is complete, you should be able to analyze the perils that would have the greatest effect on you. As you fill out this form, think about the things in your area that could force you to evacuate. What kind of freight is shipped near you? What kind of factories are there? Would your geographical terrain ease or aggravate possible problems?

Locate Your Evacuation Shelter

Preparing to survive in the wilderness is not necessary. For the most part, schools, churches, National Guard armories, and other large public buildings would be used to house evacuees. An earthquake or major disaster could cause a possible exception, where buildings that would normally be used to shelter disaster victims would be considered unsafe. Evacuees would then need to stay in tents or makeshift shelters outside. It could require time to bring in large tents for public use.

An essential part of practical preparation should be to contact relatives and friends who live nearby, yet away from your immediate area. Make arrangements to stay with them in case there is some reason for an extended evacuation during which your home might be rendered uninhabitable for several weeks or longer. Plan your escape routes on paper now. Assess neighboring areas to see what churches, armories, schools, and other buildings might be used as evacuation shelters in your area. To determine what buildings are designated as evacuation centers, call your local emergency services office, sheriff's department, police department, or Red Cross director. Don't be discouraged, however, if no one has any idea of what you are talking about.

You can calm some of your fears by going outside your immediate neighborhood and looking for churches with large gymnasiums or recreation rooms, National Guard armories, schools and colleges with gymnasiums, or buildings such as fraternal lodges with kitchen facilities and large recreation rooms. These are the kinds of buildings that would normally be used to set up evacuation centers.

In order to eliminate guesswork and confusion at the time of evacuation, buy or draw a large map of your area. Using the results and information from your completed Neighborhood Evaluation form, mark the routes to several of the buildings you or Emergency Services have determined to be the most logical evacuation centers. Be sure to record street address numbers. At all times, keep this map with your seventy-two-hour evacuation kit!

Lag Time

Most people evacuated from their homes do not expect to be away for more than one day. This is a serious misconception. Many evacuation periods last several days or more. For the first hours or even days of an emergency, you alone may have to provide your own food, clothing, and other supplies until help arrives. This period between the actual occurrence of the emergency and when help comes is known as *lag time*.

Research has shown that in most serious situations, the lag time is seventy-two hours—three days. During that time, evacuees could be faced with living in fairly primitive conditions. They may have no clean water, heat, lights, toilet facilities, or shelter.

One Utah Red Cross director noted: "Lag time is not given the emphasis that it should be given. It is one of the most critical factors during an evacuation, yet most people don't even recognize it, let alone prepare for it."

Preparation for lag time is a must. Most evacuees have not prepared at all. They simply lock their doors behind them and leave. Most of them survive the displacement, but they enjoy little dignity or comfort during the experience.

When people have prepared for evacuation, they have far fewer problems than they would have had. They are more comfortable, have activities to occupy their time, are less concerned about unfinished business, and are less likely to become a problem at a shelter.

Don't be caught unprepared! This book will show you how to get ready for a seventy-two-hour evacuation and existence in a shelter so that you will not only survive it, but survive it with a minimum of discomfort and fear.

CHAPTER TWO

THE SEVENTY-TWO HOUR EVACUATION KIT

The first and most important thing to do in preparing for an evacuation is to assemble a seventy-two-hour emergency kit for each member of your family. The emergency kits should contain basically what you will need to survive for seventy-two hours, including food and clothing. These kits must be ready and accessible *before* an evacuation order comes, and how well you prepare them will determine how well you survive a crisis with some degree of dignity and confidence if you are forced to evacuate your home.

What should you include in the kits? There is no ideal list that will fit everyone. What you include will depend on your specific needs. A thorough assessment of essentials weighed against the limitations of space will usually be the deciding factor. This book will provide some recommendations for you to consider.

You should take into account each person's particular needs, such as age, size, health, and strength. For example, kits for very young children should not include such potentially dangerous items as matches, heat tabs, fuel, pocketknives, first-aid kits, and scissors.

Consider carefully how much each kit will weigh and whether or not the person will be able to carry it without too much trouble. You never know how far or how long a kit might have to be carried.

The Container

The kind of containers you use for your kits is very important. The containers should be lightweight and compact and yet have enough room in them for the items you need. They should be sturdy enough to withstand rough handling and adverse conditions. They should have sturdy handles. If possible, they should be waterproof. However, don't wait to start assembling your kits until you have perfect containers. Start now with whatever you have—polyethylene buckets with tight-fitting lids, suitcases, or even cardboard boxes. You can always improve your kits later. Don't try to cram supplies for your entire family into one large container. If you do, you may not be able to move it when a critical situation arises. The contents of a seventy-two-hour kit should be limited to two people at the most. One is preferable.

I started my first emergency kit in a large wooden footlocker, complete with heavy rope handles and a metal hasp. I regularly accumulated supplies in this box, and from time to time I would lift the lid and gaze at the contents, enjoying the feeling of security it gave me. Then one day we decided to have an evacuation drill. When it came time to move the footlocker, I couldn't even budge it. In fact, it was so heavy that I probably couldn't have moved it even if it had been on wheels. We quickly learned that we needed to have a smaller, separate container for each member of our family.

There are several kinds of containers you might use for your emergency kits. We will consider each of them here.

Polyethylene buckets. Polyethylene buckets, in my opinion, are the best choice for a seventy-two-hour kit. A six-gallon bucket with a sturdy handle and a snug lid is almost perfect. It is large enough to contain all the essential items for one adult. It is waterproof and can be used for a washbasin or toilet. It can also be used to carry water, and it stacks well when not in use. Finally, it is inexpensive.

Backpacks. Backpacks make good containers for an emergency kit. They are easy to carry, and some are water-repellent. Pack size and style should be adapted for the individual. If used with backpacking frames, they can be used to carry sleeping bags. They do have some problems, however. They are difficult to store, and mice or weevil may be able to get into them to eat your food supplies.

Duffel bags. A good, shoulder-strap-style duffel bag

makes a fairly good emergency-kit container. Some are water-repellent, and they are quite sturdy. However, the drawstring-style bags are cumbersome, and any duffel bag is an easy target for mice or weevil.

Suitcases. Suitcases come in various sizes and stack well, but if you use them, make sure that their handles are secure. Again, mice and weevil can penetrate them easily, and they are not water-repellent. It may be possible to store items in untreated plastic trash bags inside suitcases to help keep out water.

Totebags. Totebags can be used for emergency kits if they can be closed securely, although they are usually not very sturdy. If you use a totebag, make sure that the handles are securely fastened to the bag. A totebag might be used for a child's kit.

Produce box. A sturdy waxed produce box with "handle holes" can be used as a makeshift kit container, but you should replace it with a better container as soon as possible. Such a box is not water-repellent. Placing contents in an untreated plastic trash bag would provide some protection against water.

Trunks, footlockers, and ammunition boxes. I do not recommend using these for emergency kits. They are much too heavy and unmanageable for one person to move. Also, their lids may not fit securely.

Garbage cans. Metal, plastic, or rubber garbage cans do not make good containers for emergency kits. They become much too heavy and unwieldy. Many people have recommended using them, but a thirty-gallon can full of supplies can weigh up to 200 pounds, requiring a hand truck to move it. Does that sound like something you would like to carry when the flood waters are coming?

Keep Your Kits Accessible

On a wet winter night in 1984, some friends of ours heard sirens. Suddenly a policeman pounded on their door. "You have just five minutes to get out," he said. "There is a fire in the chemical plant just west of here. Grab your family and leave." Acrid smoke was already beginning to fill the air. They picked up their children, wrapped them in quilts, jumped in the car, and drove off. They wanted to take their emergency kits, but the kits were stored under the stairs in the basement, with other objects stored on top of the kits. Unfortunately, there wasn't time to dig the kits out.

Don't let this happen to you. Keep your kits where you can grab them at a moment's notice. Find an unobtrusive yet safe and convenient spot. I use buckets for our family's kits, and I keep them stacked in a closet near our front door. One family I know have their kits in backpacks, which they hang on hooks near their back door. A widowed senior citizen I know keeps her suitcase kit in a small space at the end of a kitchen cupboard.

Label Your Kits

Be sure to label your kits with your name, address, and phone number. Use indelible marking pens, and make the writing as bright, permanent, and easily identifiable as possible. This will help you to keep track of your kits in an evacuation center, where many people could have kits similar to yours.

You might even decorate your kits for easy identification. This could also help brighten a dreary evacuation center. You may wish to use a slogan, such as "This too shall pass." Don't underestimate the positive psychological influence this can have on you and others.

It would probably be wise to label the items in your kit as well. In the long run it could prevent confusion and loss of property in a crowded shelter.

Maintain Your Kits

It would be a mistake to store your kits away and then never look at them again. Food and clothing will attract moths, weevil, and mice. Some of these pests can get through almost any kind of container. Also, watch out for mold, mildew, and rust. Avoid storing your kits in a very warm place; heat leads to rapid deterioration. Try not to store your kits on a concrete floor. Concrete "sweats." This could cause deterioration and weakening of your kit container, and eventually the items inside. Keep your kits in a dark, dry, and cool place if possible..

Your kits will not do you much good if they have been ruined through neglect. Mark a date on your calendar every six months to check them. Just a few minutes of maintenance twice a year could be the determining factor in whether or not the kits will be any good if you ever need them.

CHAPTER THREE

FOOD

During a crisis, what you eat is unusually important. You will be under more stress than usual, and you will need lots of energy, so the food you put into your emergency kit should be very high in calories. Of course, good nutrition is important too, but calorie content is the most important factor in short-term survival.

People can live for several days without food if they have water to drink. However, most of us are accustomed to regular meals and plenty of food. Trying to get through an emergency without eating would only compound the difficulties of the evacuation. And failure to provide proper nourishment for yourself would increase someone else's burden.

Besides providing nourishment, the eating of "meals" during an emergency has a positive psychological effect. It brings some order to an otherwise chaotic day, and it helps people feel that they do have some control over a difficult situation.

Of course, food may be provided in an evacuation center during an emergency, but there may be some lag time before that food is available. Also, food in an evacuation center is usually donated by individuals, restaurants, and canneries. This presents a problem for diabetics, hyperglycemics, and others with dietary restrictions. Infants and small children may not be able to eat this food either. Nursing mothers should consider the possibility that because of stress, they might not be able to produce enough milk for their babies. Several Red Cross directors have emphasized that one of the greatest problems in a major crisis, involving several days and many people, is trying to feed babies and small children.

As you prepare your emergency kits, take into account the special dietary needs and likes of your family. Try to include food that they will enjoy, that will be high in calories, and that will provide adequate nutrition. Foods that are lightweight and compact and that require no refrigeration, preparation, or cooking are best suited for an evacuation kit. Concentrated foods, such as high-energy trail bars, are good choices. Foods associated with home storage, such as grains, beans, and flour, are *not* good choices for emergency kits. They are bulky and require too much preparation. Also, an evacuation shelter is not a good place to try new, unusual foods. Stick to simple foods that your family already likes. However, nutritious staple items you already have on hand may not work in a seventy-two-hour kit! The circumstances of the evacuation as well as the space in the container are extremely limiting factors.

Foods Suitable for Evacuation Kits

You will be surprised at the wide variety of foods that are suitable for emergency kits. Many of them are available at your local supermarket. Others may be available at sporting-goods outlets, health-food stores, or food-storage supply houses.

Compressed food bars. Compressed food bars, such as granola bars and trail bars, are excellent for use in emergency kits. They store well, are lightweight, taste good, and are nutritious and high in calories.

Trail mix. Trail mixes are mixtures of such ingredients as granola, nuts, seeds, and dried fruits. They taste good, and they are high in calories and nutrition. If stored for a very long time, trail mixes can become rancid.

Dried foods. Dried foods, especially meat and fruit, are fine for seventy-two-hour kits. They taste good, are nutritious, and are satisfying. One problem with dried foods is that they may make you thirsty. This is especially true with salted jerky.

Freeze-dried foods. Freeze-dried foods are excellent additions to seventy-two-hour kits. You may be familiar with these as backpacking foods. Many are available in supermarkets, as well. They are lightweight and tasty, but water is needed for their reconstitution. If necessary, they can be reconstituted with cold water. Some freeze-dried foods come in #2 cans, but these are rather bulky for emergency kits. Freeze-dried foods tend to be higher priced than other foods.

Instant meals. You might include such "instant" meals as cups of noodles, cups of casserole, and so on. These "meals" are usually freeze-dried and will reconstitute immediately with hot water. In dire straits, cold water will work. They are an excellent consideration for seventy-two-hour kits.

Stress Foods. Such foods as hard candy, chocolate, energy bars, and sugared dry cereal are known as stress foods. These are a necessity in a seventy-two-hour kit. In stressful situations, people require an increased caloric intake to meet the extraordinary demands for energy. Stress foods meet the requirements for survival, not for a balanced diet. They are small and compact and should be liberally tucked into small spaces throughout your evacuation kit. They also help boost morale. If you can't eat sugar because of dietary restrictions, try the diabetic candies made with honey or other ingredients.

Snack-sized canned goods. Snack-sized canned goods make good additions to evacuation kits if they have pull-top lids or twist-open keys. You should consider such items as corned beef, deviled ham, vienna sausages, luncheon meat, pork and beans, tuna, single-serving soup, pudding, and fruit. The "flat size" (approximately 6 ounces) of foods such as chicken or pineapple works well as long as an opener is part of the equipment.

Snack foods. Some snack foods work well in evacuation kits because of their packaging. Snack-pack cheese and crackers, snack-pack peanut butter and crackers, roasted nuts in cellophane or foil packages, or small variety-pack dry or sugared cereals are a few examples.

Drink mixes. Drink mixes add variety to a seventy-two-hour kit. Try such items as hot chocolate mix, instant breakfast mixes, and presweetened powdered fruit drinks. These usually come in foil envelopes, so they fit easily in the kit.

Liquid beverages. Beverages are now available in many kinds of handy packages, including foil packets and foil-lined boxes (a straw comes with them). These are perfect for use in emergency kits. Most of them are aseptic and so will keep for a long time. Because of the processing no refrigeration is required. Shelf life is not indefinite—but it is long. Juices and even milk are available. You might also consider using small cans of juice that open with a pull tab.

A Seventy-two-Hour Menu

Following is a sample menu that could get one person through a seventy-two-hour emergency. Although it lacks the bulk of usual meals; it contains a good variety of food with sufficient calories, and it is fairly inexpensive. Note that although liquid is not shown in this menu, you must keep it in mind as you plan!

Item		Calories	Approximate Amount for 72 Hours	Approximate Calories
Granola milk bar	9 oz.	230	3	690
Chewy granola bar	8 oz.	130	3	390
Dried apples	3 oz.	275	12 oz.	1100
Dried raisins	3 oz.	289	12 oz.	1156
Salted peanuts	3 oz.	585	9 oz.	1795
Instant breakfast	2 envelopes	130	6 envelopes	780
Protein energy bar	1.4 oz.	160	6	960
			Total:	6871 ÷ 3 days = 2290.33 calories per day

Foods Not Suitable for Evacuation Kits

The following kinds of food are not suitable for seventy-two-hour kits.

Commercially dehydrated foods. Commercially dehydrated foods require a great deal of water for reconstitution, and they are difficult to prepare. These foods cannot be eaten as if they were dried foods. They must be reconstituted.

Bottled foods. Bottled foods are too heavy and take up too much space to make them practical for emergency kits. Also, bottled foods break easily.

Commercially canned foods. Other than the small snack-sized canned goods, commercially canned foods weigh too much and take up too much space. One government agency published a list of canned goods that they felt should be put in an evacuation kit. For two people, the weight of the cans was fifty-five pounds! This is just not practical. You might use canned goods to get started on your kits, but if you do, you should replace them with more compact foods as soon as possible. Don't forget to include a can opener.

Whole grains, beans, pasta. Do not even consider such foods as grains, beans, or pasta. Preparing these foods in the trying circumstances of an evacuation shelter would be almost impossible.

Food for a Baby or Toddler

If you have a baby or toddler, you will need to provide for his special needs. If you are a nursing mother, you should include some liquid formula in your kit in case you are unable to nurse because of tension and shock. Even though powdered formula weighs less, you may not be able to use it if water is not available. You may want to include both liquid and powdered formula in your kit. How much should you include? You will need to estimate how much your baby will be drinking six months from now. If your baby is allergic to milk, you will need to include a soy-based or other kind of formula. You could also include sterile bottled juices.

If your baby is a little older or is a toddler, you will need to include some kind of baby food. A baby probably will *not* be able to eat from an adult's kit. There are many instant foods you could use—cereal, fruits, and vegetables are all available. These must be reconstituted with water, but even cold water would do in a pinch. Whatever you use, be sure that they are foods your child has eaten before and likes.

Containers, Utensils, and Equipment

You will probably need to include some kind of utensils or other equipment in your kits, and probably some of your food will need to be stored in small containers. You should try to use as few of these items as possible, as they take up space that could be used for food, and they add weight. The kinds of food you have chosen will directly affect what equipment you will need.

Some small containers for storing food in seventy-two-hour kits include small cans with tight-fitting lids, such as peanut cans, chip-dip cans, and so on. Small glass jars with twist-on lids may be all right, but they can be broken. You can also use small plastic freezer containers. Sturdy sandwich or freezer bags might work, but mice and weevil can get into them. Do not use aluminum foil or paper bags as containers in your kits.

Equipment and utensils you might consider are:

small cooking pots
spoons, forks, and knives (some plastic, some metal)
Sierra cups (metal cups that you can heat food in or
    drink from)
mess kits (Scout mess kits work well)
napkins or paper towels
small bottle of dish soap
hot pad (a wash cloth can serve a dual purpose)
can opener (the GI type works well)
matches in waterproof container
small backpacking stove with fuel
canned heat and folding stove
heat tablets and winged-tab stove or folding stove

The extremely small winged-tab or folding stoves that use heat tabs are best suited for a seventy-two-hour kit.

Small backpacking stoves that use liquid fuel also work although they weigh more and take up more space.

Planning Your Kit

Use the worksheets on pages 48-55 to help you plan what food and equipment to buy and include in your kits. They will help you plan for your individual needs and to obtain the best prices for what you buy. Use these worksheets as a reference to help you adjust and refine your kits until they are exactly what you need.

Work in pencil, not pen, so that you can make adjustments as you go. Involve everyone in your family in the planning. This will help them understand how to cope with an evacuation, and it will help them become familiar with the contents of their kits.

After you have read this book, using the worksheets it contains and making notes in the margins, put it in the top of your evacuation kit, where it will be a valuable resource as you update your kits or if you ever need to evacuate.

Begin with what you have! You can always improve your kit later, but any preparation is better than none. Also, if you can't afford to purchase all the items you need now, buy just a few things each payday until your kits are completed.

Practice Sessions

Before a critical situation forces you from home, it is important to practice preparing and eating meals from the kind of food you have included in your evacuation kits. A meal for one person might consist entirely of a granola bar, three graham crackers, half a cup of raisins, and a hot drink from a mix. You may want to find out what a normally hot food tastes like prepared with cold water. A practice session might seem more real if it is held outside your home. Also, no one should be able to go home and eat some more after the practice session. As your family eats, you will quickly learn what tastes good and what doesn't and what works and what doesn't. This will help you make adjustments in what you include in your kits.

If you are including a small folding stove in your kits, try cooking your meal on it. This will help you learn how to use the stove before you have to do it in an emergency. Every member of your family should be taught safety precautions in using the stove. For example, the instant a lit match touches a heat tab, the tab will ignite, although you may not be able to see it burning. A person not aware of this could easily be burned. Be sure to put the stove on a stable, level surface.

Holding a practice session with household members is one of the most important parts of gaining realistic understanding and experience of what it means to prepare meals with food and equipment in your kit.

CHAPTER FOUR

WATER

During an evacuation, water may or may not be available. Usually, water can be found at an evacuation shelter, but there may be lag time until water becomes available. Also, community water supplies may have become polluted; this is a common occurrence after an earthquake. If electrical power is out, the pumps that ordinarily bring water through the system may not be working. After the Mexico City earthquake of 1985, it took two days to get water into some areas.

Because water may not be immediately available at an evacuation center, you should plan to carry some water with you. The minimum amount of drinking water for one person for seventy-two hours is six quarts. This much water weighs twelve pounds. Other needs, such as brushing teeth and preparing food, usually require an additional two gallons a day.

As you decide how much water to carry with you, consider the number of people in your family and their ages, health, and strength. Teenagers, for example, may require more water than other family members. Realistically, how much water *can* you carry?

One advantage to keeping your kits in polyethylene buckets is that you can use the buckets to carry water that might be available at an evacuation center or from other community sources. If you are carrying some canned goods in your kits, you may not need to carry as much water. A #303 can of fruit, for example, contains about a cup of liquid. And if you are carrying some packaged liquid beverages, you will not need as much water to drink. If many of your foods are dried, salty, or spicy, or if they require water for reconstitution or preparation, you will need more water than usual.

Water Containers

In most cases, water containers will be carried outside your kits. Many kinds of containers can be used to carry water. Some of the best are Scout canteens, which come with a strap for carrying, and backpacking flasks, which usually hook onto a belt. Other possible containers include quart-sized plastic soda-pop bottles (replace with better containers as soon as you can), two-and-a-half-gallon or five-gallon water jugs, and sturdy quart or half-gallon milk bottles (replace as soon as you can). Whatever you use, make sure it is clean, has a tight-fitting lid, and was designed for food or water.

Fill your containers as full as you can, eliminating all the air possible. This will help reduce the growth of bacteria. Of course, if there is danger that your water will freeze, you will have to allow some space for the water to expand. Otherwise, your containers could break and leak, ruining the contents of your kits.

Water bottles could be attached to belts for easier carrying, although belts made of rope may be uncomfortable. Nylon rope could be used to lash several containers together, creating a handle, or containers could be tied to a polyethylene bucket or backpack. You could also fashion a yoke to wear over your shoulders for carrying water bottles.

By using the worksheets on pages 52-55 you will be able to figure out the amount of water you need, as well as the number and kinds of containers necessary for your kits.

Purifying Water

No matter how much water you decide to carry with you, you should know how to purify it. It may have become contaminated with age. Also, water at a shelter may have become contaminated. If water is cloudy or polluted, it should be purified before use. If the water is clear but you are not sure whether it is safe or not, purify it anyway. It could contain bacteria, and it is better to be safe than sorry.

You should have the following water-purification supplies in your emergency kits:

a collapsible bucket (if your kits are not in polyethylene buckets) or sturdy plastic bags. (Use only food-grade

plastic bags. Colored or treated trash bags will not
do, nor will bread sacks or very thin plastic bags.)
a small pan in which to boil water
cheesecloth or other cloth for straining impurities from
    water
heat tabs or other heat source
water purification tablets, tincture of iodine, or liquid
chlorine bleach

If water is especially dirty, strain it through a cloth to remove debris and dirt. Then boil it for three to five minutes
to kill bacteria. This is the safest way to purify water. Let
the water cool before drinking it. Be sure to take into account the high rate of evaporation at the boiling point and
increase the amount you boil. Otherwise, the water could
boil away, leaving less than the amount needed. This may
seem like a trivial point, but it could compound the stress
and problems of an already difficult situation. Boiled water
will taste better if you pour it from one container to another
a few times to put oxygen back into it. This is also true of
water that has been stored for some time. To use water purification tablets, follow the instructions on the package.
Usually, four tablets a gallon are sufficient. Use twelve
drops of tincture of iodine or eight drops of chlorine bleach
to purify a gallon of water. Mix the tablets, iodine, or bleach
thoroughly into the water and let it stand for several minutes. If the water is cloudy, double the number of tablets or
drops of iodine or bleach. The water will taste better if you
let it stand for a little while before drinking it.

CHAPTER FIVE

SHELTER, CLOTHING, HEAT, AND LIGHT

During an evacuation, you will almost certainly be directed to stay in an evacuation center, such as a school, a church, or an armory. You will probably be in a large room with a concrete or wooden floor and brick walls—not a very comfortable or private place. So, to make yourself as comfortable as possible, you will want to include in your evacuation kits some form of shelter (mostly for privacy), clothing, and sources of warmth and light (there may be no electricity).

Shelter

Perhaps the best shelter to use in an evacuation center is a small, lightweight tube tent. You should consider this to be an essential piece of equipment for each kit you put together (except those for babies or toddlers). They are relatively inexpensive and can be purchased almost anywhere. Other possibilities are backpacking tents, plastic or nylon tarps with ropes to suspend them, or even plastic ground covers. If you have tents that you use for camping, you may be able to use them during an evacuation.

Blankets

If you are evacuated to a public shelter, a critical part of your seventy-two-hour kits will be some kind of blanket for each member of your family. Blankets provide warmth and give a feeling of security. A blanket can also be used as a screen to provide some measure of privacy in a crowded evacuation center. This is especially important if you have to use some kind of makeshift toilet. As you evaluate the kinds of blankets you might use, consider those you already have on hand. The major problem with most blankets is how to get them to fit inside a kit. As soon as possible, obtain a blanket that fits *inside* with all other items as well, to keep the seventy-two-hour kit compact and manageable.

Wool blankets. Wool blankets are very warm, even when wet. However, they are bulky and weigh a lot, and they take a long time to dry.

Virgin acrylic blankets. Virgin acrylic blankets are very warm, have many of the advantages of wool, and yet are lightweight and "squishable." A twin-size blanket will fit nicely into a six-gallon bucket with all the other supplies. These blankets also dry quickly. This is probably the best blanket for an evacuation kit.

Thermal blankets. Thermal blankets are warm, but they are heavy and bulky.

Polyester/acrylic blankets. Polyester/acrylic blankets are fairly warm, but they are not as warm as some other blankets. They are also fairly heavy and bulky.

Quilts and comforters. Quilts and comforters are very warm, but they weigh a lot, are bulky, and take a long time to dry.

Sleeping bags. Sleeping bags are very warm, and many are waterproof. If your kit container is a backpack with a frame, you can easily carry a sleeping bag with it. They are bulky, though, and do not dry quickly.

Backpacking sleeping bags. Most backpacking sleeping bags are extremely warm and waterproof, and they are usually lightweight though bulky. They do not dry quickly.

Emergency blankets and space blankets. These blankets are usually made out of foil or paper. They give some warmth and are very compact and lightweight. They do not really feel like a blanket, however, and they will not hold up under heavy use.

Baby blankets. Large or crib-size baby blankets are warm and are smaller than regular blankets. They should dry quickly.

Blankets cut in half or blanket material remnants. You can take advantage of a twin-size blanket (or blanket material) yet still have a blanket compact enough to fit into a kit by cutting a larger blanket in half and sewing the edges to prevent fraying. It will still have bulk, but not nearly as much.

Heat

Usually it is not practical to carry a heat source in an evacuation kit. The small folding stoves used for cooking give off some heat. Any heat source would have to be small, compact, and lightweight, as well as functional. The most practical solution is to use the same source you will be using to cook with. Carefully evaluate your needs, your climate, and the problems you might be faced with; then determine whether or not you should consider some kind of stove for heat. In a seventy-two-hour kit, even the lightweight backpacking equipment is almost too bulky. And this difficulty is compounded with the weight and volume of fuel that would be needed. In most instances, you will be evacuated to a shelter, but lag time could be a problem if you live in an area with cold winters. Be sure to include matches in your kits.

Light

You should provide a source of light for every member of your family, keeping in mind the constant limitations of space and weight. Following are some light sources for you to consider.

Flashlights. Flashlights are excellent sources of light. They are safe and lightweight, and with new batteries and bulb, they will provide about seven hours of light. Include an extra set of batteries with each flashlight. It is recommended that every kit contain a working flashlight (except a baby's or toddler's). Pack it as one of the top items in the kit!

Candles. Small utility or camping candles may be used in emergency kits, but avoid using the longer dinner candles, which do not burn as long. The use of candles requires close adult supervision! If you are going to use candles, you would be wise to put them in candle lanterns, which will help support the candles solidly. Or small, solid candle holders may be used for the same purpose.

Backpacking lanterns. Backpacking lanterns are small, lightweight lanterns that burn liquid fuel. Some are collapsible. Consider the weight and bulk of additional fuel.

Fluorescent lanterns. Fluorescent lanterns burn brighter and longer than a regular flashlight, but they are also larger and weigh more.

Chemical light sticks. Chemical light sticks are small and lightweight, and most last about thirty minutes. Some last up to twelve hours. Their light is not bright, and once they are lit, they cannot be turned off. They continue to burn until they are used up. They cannot be used again. Also, they are fairly expensive. Each person would need several of them. They are not recommended as the only source of light for a seventy-two-hour kit.

If you decide to use any light source that requires fuel or flame, supervise its use carefully, and set up some safety rules for your family. Be especially cautious around children and in crowded places.

It is particularly important that you hold practice sessions so that the realities of functioning with your light sources are understood.

Clothing

You should include one *complete* change of clothing in your evacuation kits for each member of your family. You can probably use clothing that you already have on hand, but you should make sure that it is good, sturdy clothing rather than playclothes, lightweight casual clothing, or worn-out clothing. Don't worry much about color coordination or style. The object is to keep your body warm, protected, and dry. Remember that you may be exposed to the elements and to the public, and you will probably be engaged in helping people and in doing hard work. Your clothes will need to withstand the strain.

Depending on your climate, you may want to keep a list of one set of clothing for summer and one for winter and then put the appropriate set into your seventy-two-hour kits every six months. There isn't room in a kit for heavy winter coats, hats, and gloves, but in an evacuation there is usually time to open the closet and put on these items if you need them.

But more important than excess weight is that the wrong kind of clothing in weather extremes will compound already severe problems. Lightweight, thin summer clothes in the dead of winter—or in chilling, freezing rain—would turn a minor crisis into a disaster. Heavy wools, sweaters, scarves, and gloves in the middle of a heat wave would be just as serious. This point must be taken seriously, especially if you are dealing with babies, the elderly, or the ill.

Remember to take into consideration individual needs. For example, for many people support hose are a necessity, not a luxury. Don't forget such things as neck braces, dentures, glasses, and arch supports.

One item of clothing that should be in every kit you prepare is a poncho. A poncho is versatile—it gives protection from the weather, it can provide shade on a hot day, and it increases your ability to stay warm. You and your family should try wearing your ponchos before you actually have to. This is especially important for teenagers, who are so style conscious. Teach them that a poncho is to help them be more comfortable, not to help them look stylish. The poncho is one of the items that should be packed at the top of your kit.

Clothes for a Baby or Toddler

In providing clothes for a baby or toddler, think large. Six months from now, your child may have grown a great deal, so the clothing you include in his kit should account for that. A medium-weight, stretchable, terry-cloth play suit should work well, and it wouldn't matter if it was quite a bit too large. Shoes may be impractical, but T-shirts and socks are a must! Blanket sleepers might be used instead of a blanket, and you can always remove a baby's clothing if it becomes too warm. The kit for a baby or small child will need more consistent review and evaluation than any of the others. It may seem like busywork, but it could make the difference between chaos or "only" a challenge in the unsettled conditions of a shelter.

Be sure to keep a large box (with handle) of disposable diapers on hand. Cloth diapers will not do, because you will have no practical way to wash or store them once they have been used. Don't try to repack diapers into a kit; they are too bulky. If you live in a wet climate, you may want to repack them into a heavy plastic garbage bag to keep out moisture. Some of these heavy-duty trash bags now have handles, which would help in carrying. A good thing to include in a baby's kit is a package of premoistened babies' wipe-up towelettes. Also, don't forget to include a pacifier and perhaps a small rattle or toy. Because of rapid growth, dietary changes, and other continually changing requirements, a kit for a baby or toddler is one of the most difficult to assemble. Another option would be to methodically create a small child's seventy-two-hour kit on paper. It is essential that you complete this "paper kit" while you have a clear mind and can reason out the items that will be needed. During an evacuation, you could have difficulty remembering such details, particularly if you have more than one small child. If your child has a "security blanket" or favorite teddy bear, be sure to include it on the list. If everyone else's kit is ready, you will probably have time to gather a baby's kit following your list. Of course, it would be logical to have a container and as many spare items as possible already gathered. Periodically review and update your "paper kit." Make sure you keep it with your other seventy-two-hour kits.

Also, check your child's actual kit frequently to make sure that he has not outgrown the clothing in it and that the other items in the kit will still meet his needs.

CHAPTER SIX

SANITATION AND FIRST AID

One of the most overlooked and underestimated problems during the turmoil of establishing an evacuation shelter is the lack of sanitation. Usually an evacuation center will have toilet facilities, but if water supplies are cut off or rationed, you will need to have other arrangements. In some instances portable chemical toilets may be brought in. But during the lag time you must be able to cope with the situation!

Adequate toilet facilites are especially important during an unsettled shelter situation because stress, a change of diet, lack of privacy, and loss of security compound to upset the digestive system. Good judgment, a sense of humor, and, most of all, advance preparation will help solve sanitation problems.

One important reason to use a polyethylene bucket for at least one of your seventy-two-hour kits is that it can be used as a makeshift toilet. To do this, you will need a roll of toilet paper (it can be smashed flat to fit into your kit), some heavy trash bags with wire ties, large rubber bands (at least a quarter-inch wide), and a small bottle of disinfectant (such as chlorine bleach, Lysol, or PineSol).

Insert a garbage sack into the empty bucket with the edge folded down over the top of the bucket. Secure it in place with a large rubber band. After using this toilet, put some disinfectant into the bag and cover the bucket with its lid. This toilet can be used several times. To dispose of the waste, remove the rubber band, twist the bag closed, and secure it tightly with a wire tie. Finally, remove the bag from the bucket. An officer at an evacuation center can tell you how to dispose of the bag.

You should have your whole family practice sitting on your makeshift toilet to get a feel for the balance required. This will help diminish problems and maintain dignity if you ever have to use it.

You can obtain some privacy while using this toilet by

having family members hold a blanket in front of it, or you could suspend a blanket on a rope in front of it.

Personal Hygiene

If, during an evacuation, you are exposed to mud, sewage, or other forms of pollution, it is a necessity to be able to get clean.

As much as possible, you should maintain good hygiene while staying in a shelter. You can brush your teeth, wash your face, comb your hair, and even wash your body with a wet washcloth. This will prevent the spread of disease and irritation, which only increase the stress of evacuation.

Doing such things as brushing your teeth at a routine time also brings some order to the day and has a healthy psychological effect.

Some items you should include in your kits for personal hygiene include the following:

a bar of soap
a small bottle of shampoo
toothbrush and small tube of toothpaste
small mirror
a comb or brush
a washcloth and small towel
disposable razors/shaving gear
premoistened towelettes
a small bottle of deodorant
feminine hygiene supplies
denture or contact lens requirements
other individual needs

First Aid

In your seventy-two-hour kit, you should be sure to include a small and simple first-aid kit for treating minor injuries and ailments, which could otherwise become serious if left for a few days. Be sure that your kit contains a first-aid manual, and read it before you pack it away. Know what supplies are in your first-aid kit, and be sure you know how to use them.

A small commercial first-aid kit works well. If you would rather assemble your own kit, contact your pharmacist or the Red Cross for suggestions about what to put in it. What you include will depend upon the needs of your family and your budget. The Red Cross publishes excellent first-aid manuals and provides classes in first aid. At least one member of your family should attend one of these classes, if possible.

Following are some items you might want to include in a first-aid kit:

aspirin or nonaspirin pain reliever
hydrogen peroxide or other antiseptic
cotton balls or swabs
burn ointment
adhesive-strip bandages
gauze
a needle
elastic bandages
sterile bandages
matches (for sterilizing)
scissors
safety pins (in assorted sizes)
petroleum jelly
tweezers
adhesive tape

If you have a baby, you should also consider including liquid pain reliever, teething ointment, diaper-rash ointment, baby oil, and whatever else your baby may need.

People commonly arrive at an evacuation center without the prescription medicine they have to take. If you require prescription medicine or allergy medicine, save yourself future problems by planning ahead now! If at all possible to *safely* do so, keep a prescription with your kit. Ask your doctor or pharmacist for specific instructions about how to do so.

CHAPTER SEVEN

MISCELLANEOUS ITEMS

During the summer of 1984, a fast-moving canyon fire forced residents of Malibu, California, to evacuate. According to one newspaper account, a well-known Hollywood personality ran frantically from room to room trying to decide what to take with her, but she had only forty-five minutes to decide, and she had made no preparations for such an emergency. First she gathered her valuable paintings into the middle of her living room, but then she remembered other valuables and went to get them. The forty-five minutes passed quickly, and finally she was forced to leave her home without taking anything.

You should decide now, before a disaster, what you will do with your treasures in case of an emergency. If you have large paintings, you may have to leave them hanging on your wall. If you have time, you might be able to put them in a safe place somewhere inside your house. What about such irreplaceable items as photo albums, scrapbooks, or heirlooms? If you make plans now about what to do with these things, you may save valuables that would otherwise be lost forever through panic and indecision.

Important Documents

Every family has important documents that need to be preserved. These include deeds; wills; insurance policies; birth, marriage, and death certificates; and so on. For many families, it is difficult to find a particular document even during normal times. And it would be almost impossible for them to gather up all their important papers in an emergency. Also, many people have more than enough important papers to fill an entire emergency kit. There is little semblance of order during an evacuation. In the confusion and possibility of relocation there is a good chance papers could be lost or inadvertently taken. The possibility of loss or destruction increases with the severity and length of the crisis. A public evacuation shelter or tube tent is obviously not a secure place to keep important documents, so don't try to take documents with you.

The best way to protect your important documents is to make several good copies of them. Have these copies notarized, if it will make them more valid in your area. Then put the originals in a safety deposit box at your bank, file a copy at home, and give a copy in a clearly marked, sealed envelope to a friend or relative who lives *outside* your area. Some of these documents could be required to insure your rights, to prove ownership, and to file claims in case your home is destroyed.

Be sure to check your papers regularly to make sure that they are always up to date.

Following is a list of documents that you may need to protect:

Social Security cards and records
deeds
insurance policies
stocks and bonds
wills
savings and checking account numbers and locations
credit card numbers and companies
immunization records
birth, marriage, and death records
inventory of household goods—photographic, if possible
financial records
personal and family records, certificates, and journals

Money

In addition to items you will want to leave in a safe place at home, there are a number of miscellaneous items you will want to take with you. One of these is money. Even during a crisis, you may need some money for such small things as telephone calls or a tankful of gas. Don't forget to take your wallet or purse as you walk out the door. You shouldn't need a lot of money, and your checkbook and emergency credit card should allow you to make larger purchases if you need to.

It would be foolish to try to carry large amounts of money, jewelry, or other valuables with you to an evacuation shelter, especially since these could be lost quite easily. Let common sense be your guide, and keep in mind the size and needs of your family.

Morale Boosters

During their stay in an evacuation center, people often become discouraged and bored. Children become restless and anxious, and so do adults. At such times, you will feel glad that you have tucked away a few small items to help boost morale. Some items you might want to include in your seventy-two-hour kits include small games, card games, pocket-size puzzle books, crayons and notepad, paperback books, a few small pencils, small copies of the scriptures, and perhaps some needlework.

The next time you go to the library, check out a book of party games that can be played with little or no preparation or equipment. Learn how to play a few of these and perhaps make a simple list of some of them to keep in your evacuation kit as a reminder.

A piece of candy or some treat also helps boost morale, especially for children. Include candy or treats that can double as stress foods.

Important Phone Numbers

In your kit, keep a list of names and phone numbers of people you may need to reach, such as family members, friends, and employers. There may not be a phone book at an evacuation center, and in the confusion, you may not be able to remember important numbers. With your list of phone numbers, keep a small change purse or container full of coins so you will be able to use a pay phone if you need to. Keep this near the top of your kit so you will not have to empty the rest of your kit to find it.

The Don't-Forget List

Keep a don't-forget list with each one of your kits. This list should include items that you use each day and so can't be included with your kit but that you *must* take with you. These items might include prescription medicines, eyeglasses, and so on. You must also write down the location of the items so you will be able to find them immediately, or so that if someone outside your family is helping you evacuate, he will be able to find them. Tape this list to the outside of the lid on each kit.

Other Items

There are other items that you may want to include in your kits. Here are a few for you to consider:

Scout knife or pocketknife
100 feet of one-eighth-inch nylon rope
pocket-size sewing kit
assorted safety pins
untreated plastic garbage bags (can be used as a poncho, a ground cloth, or a garbage container)
tape
small scissors
small wind-up clock
small tools (screwdriver, pliers, hammer)

CHAPTER EIGHT

COMMUNICATIONS

During the summer of 1985, a series of terrible, destructive tornadoes struck throughout the midwest. My husband and I were traveling through this area when a tornado hit. We took shelter in a hotel and watched the television all night as the Emergency Broadcast System kept us informed about the direction and intensity of the storms. They covered each county, section by section, where the tornado was. It was a frightening experience, but it was comforting to have that helpful information.

Usually during a crisis, instructions about what to do will come through the news media. According to the Civil Preparedness Agency's *Disaster Operations Manual*, it is a "widespread but erroneous idea that people are apt to panic in a threatening or dangerous situation. This hardly ever happens. People want to get solid, down-to-earth, and practical advice from their governments." Local broadcast stations, especially those with emergency power generators and equipment, can provide extensive information about disaster conditions, warnings, what to do to handle specific problems, and how to locate missing family members. They also help restore order and help people to be calm. The government's standardized Emergency Broadcast System operates throughout the nation.

To make sure you can take advantage of this information, include in each of your kits a portable, battery-powered transistor radio with an extra set of fresh batteries for each one. *This is an absolute necessity.* Keep the radios near the top of your kits so that they will be readily accessible.

Teach your family to resist the temptation to play with these radios. Before you go to an evacuation center, set up rules about how often and how long the radios may be used to play music while you have to stay there. Remember that the main purpose of the radios is to provide information and instructions about the emergency. This might be a good topic to discuss during an evacuation practice session.

In some communities, a special siren will be sounded in an emergency. These are usually tested from time to time, so you may already be familiar with their sound. If the siren gives a steady tone for three to five minutes, a peacetime emergency is occurring. If it gives a wavering tone for three to five minutes, there has been an enemy attack. In either case, you should immediately turn on your radio or television for instructions.

If the emergency is a natural disaster, such as a hurricane, flood, or tornado, the radio or television may tell you there is a *watch*. That means you will have some time to prepare for possible danger. If the station tells you that there is a *warning*, that means that the disaster has actually begun. In this case, follow the instructions that are being broadcast, and go to the safest place you can.

During an emergency warning, do not try to use your telephone to call the authorities to verify that there is an emergency or to obtain more information. Tying up the phone lines might prevent emergency calls from being made. Use the phone only if you have to.

Whatever you do, don't spread rumors. Use common sense. If you hear something from a neighbor that you are uncertain about, verify it before you pass it on. The information you give to others could affect their health, their safety, or even their lives. Sometimes, when rumors are flying, the media will say what information is only rumor. The media—not your neighbor—is your best source of information.

Another way you may learn about impending danger is from your local police or the National Guard, who may be going through your neighborhood issuing instructions through a bullhorn. If this happens, you may be in life-threatening danger, and you should follow their instructions explicitly and immediately.

CHAPTER NINE

NEIGHBORHOOD COOPERATION

In the spring of 1985, a gas leak in a certain city forced the evacuation of a ten-block area. News cameras were brought to the scene, and the first thing viewers saw was a woman trying to enter the evacuation area. Police officers held her back as she explained in anguish, "I have to get through! I left my children alone while I went to the store. The oldest one is only ten. I must get home!" Calmly yet firmly the policemen told her she could not go into the area.

An emergency will not wait to happen until everyone in your family is safely home. Chances are, it will occur when one or more members of your family are away at work, at play, or at school. In the ensuing confusion, you may not be able to get everyone together. If you have only a few minutes to evacuate, you may have no choice but to leave without someone. Also, usually no one outside the evacuation area is allowed to enter it. Family members may not be able to come home and help. What can you do in this situation?

The Care-in-a-Crisis Program

The best way to make sure that all of your family members are taken care of is to set up a Care-in-a-Crisis Program in your neighborhood. In this program, you and one or two neighbors who live near you make specific arrangements about how you will watch out for each other during an evacuation.

The first step is to decide which family or families you would like to team up with and then to invite them to meet with you to discuss the program. When you meet, give each family a copy of the form entitled "Family Information," which is printed in the back of this book. Each family should fill out this form and then give each other a copy of it. Next, give each family a copy of the form entitled "Care-in-a-Crisis Plan," which is also printed in the back of this book. You should fill out these forms together during your meeting. If necessary, you should have more than one meeting, and you should discuss who will do what in every conceivable evacuation situation. Then, write down the decisions you make on your planning forms. Emphasize that no one can afford to take anything for granted. You should plan for every contingency in specific detail.

Of course, you will be responsible for caring for your own family first, but the Care-in-a-Crisis Program gives you the added security of having someone else to turn to if the need arises.

Be sure to share your decisions with close friends or relatives who do not live in your area, so that in an emergency, they will know whom to contact, and they will also not feel that they have to endanger their own lives by coming to rescue you. In addition, you should keep copies of your plans by your telephone and in your evacuation kits. You should also inform such people as baby-sitters, day-care personnel, and nannies about your plans.

As you make your plans, you should consider others in your neighborhood who live alone or who have special health problems. Include them if you can.

At the evacuation center, too, you can continue to watch out for each other. Children can be on the buddy system, where they stay together with a partner and take care of each other. Teach your children the importance of being where they say they will be, when they say they will be. They should always let you know where they are going and when they will be back, and you should likewise keep them informed of your whereabouts. Then in an emergency, you will have less trouble finding each other and getting together according to your emergency plan.

CHAPTER TEN

EVACUATION

If you have followed the suggestions in the preceding chapters, you are prepared to survive and stay in an evacuation shelter—almost. Now you need to plan for the evacuation itself.

Transportation

In most cases, you will be able to leave your area in your own car. This is an advantage because it gives you great mobility and allows you to transport your supplies and family with ease. As a precaution, you should always keep your gas tank at least half full. Gasoline pumps do not work if the electricity is off, and during a panic, you might not be able to get to them anyway.

If you live in a large city, there could be traffic jams during an evacuation, and you should have planned your escape routes to avoid these, if possible. Plan to leave as quickly as possible so that you will not be stranded by flooded roads or fallen trees or wires. As you travel, keep listening to the radio for information and instructions, and if certain evacuation routes are specified or recommended, use them rather than trying to find shortcuts of your own. Don't try anything foolish, such as driving across a field or hazardous area. You don't want to be stranded.

If you don't have an automobile, or during the emergency can't use one, you will have to find some other method of transportation. You may be able to ride out on a motorcycle or bicycle, and you should consider obtaining a small trailer or sidecar that you can use with such vehicles to transport supplies. These vehicles could also be fitted with baskets.

Often during an evacuation, emergency planners will provide some sort of transportation, such as buses. You can also arrange with your neighbors for transportation in your Care-in-a-Crisis plans. If you live in a senior-citizen retirement complex or similar facility, you should find out what arrangements have been made for transportation by the management of your facility or by your community. If no arrangements have been made, you may be able to help organize a group to make them.

What If You Have to Walk Out?

Under some circumstances, such as a gas leak, you may be forced to walk out of the evacuation area. You and your family should plan carefully for such an eventuality, considering the age, health, and strength of your family members; the distance you might have to travel; and the weight and size of the supplies you will have to carry with you.

Almost any kind of transportation will make your journey easier if you have to walk. You can carry supplies or even children in a wagon, a wheelbarrow, a wheeled cart, or a baby buggy or stroller. One young single mother of two children who had to walk out of an area said, "I strapped my littlest child on my back, put my other child in the front of our baby stroller, set my makeshift kit on the back of the stroller, and away we went. I admit it wasn't the best, but because of the stroller I could go."

Practice Sessions

Before a disaster actually comes, practice evacuating your home, both in your automobile and on foot. Focus on the emergencies most likely to occur in your area. Make sure everyone knows how to act and what to do in each kind of emergency. Practice doing the different things. These practice drills could prove priceless when the real thing occurs. Research has shown that familiar situations lessen panic. You are more likely to keep your wits about you if you have already practiced what you may sometime be forced to do. Practice sessions will also help you to see where you need to change your plans and make adjustments.

Pets

If you have pets, find out what you should do to insure their survival. Call your local emergency services or animal control center to see if you can take your pet to an evacuation center in a pet carrier if the need arises. In some places, portable kennels have been set up outside the evacuation center. Do not simply turn your pets loose, thinking they can fend for themselves. In an emergency, officials may destroy loose animals to prevent confusion, accidents, and the spread of disease. Laws and policies about this matter may be different in different places. You should find out now what to do with your pet in case of an evacuation.

Leaving Your Home

As you leave your home, if you have time and have not received other instructions from authorities, turn down your heat or turn off your air conditioner, shut off your gas appliances, disconnect your electrical appliances (except your freezer and refrigerator), store any perishables, lock your doors and windows, and park and lock extra vehicles in your garage, carport, or driveway. The National Guard or the police usually patrol evacuated areas to prevent looting.

Returning Home

When officials say it is all right, you can return to your home, but you should not do so before that time, even if you are tempted to do so. Remember that shock, loss, and anxiety may cloud your usual good judgment. Determine now to obey official policy. It could save your life.

As you return home, continue to listen to the radio for information and instructions. This may help you avoid trouble and return home more easily. Do not attempt to visit disaster areas where rescue operations or evacuations are still going on. Doing so could only add to the trouble and confusion there.

When you get home, use extreme caution in entering or working in buildings that may have been damaged or weakened. They could collapse without warning.

Don't take lanterns, torches, or any kind of flame into a damaged building. There may be leaking gas or other flammable materials present. Use battery-powered flashlights for light. You can check for leaking gas by smell. If you smell gas, open all windows and doors and turn off the main gas valve at the meter. Don't turn on light switches or try to use the telephone, as these can produce sparks that will ignite the gas. Leave the house immediately and notify the gas company or the police. Then, don't reenter the house until an authorized person tells you it is safe to do so.

Watch out for fallen or damaged electrical wires. If you see any, notify the power company, and keep people away from them. If any of your appliances are wet, turn off the main power switch in your house. Then, unplug the wet appliance and dry it out. After that, you can plug it back in and then turn the power back on. But don't do any of these things if you are wet or if there is water in your house. If your fuses blow when the power is restored, turn off the power again and look for short circuits in your house wiring and appliances.

Check your food and water supplies before using them. Foods that require refrigeration may be spoiled if the power has been off for a long time. Do not use fresh food that has been in contact with flood water, which is usually contaminated.

Be sure to wear shoes in all areas near debris or broken glass. If your house has been damaged, check closets, shelves, and stairways carefully. Open doors slowly to avoid being hit by falling objects. Clean up any spilled medicines, cleaning products, or other potentially harmful materials.

Don't drive in the disaster area unless you absolutely have to, and then use extreme caution. Watch for road hazards, and report them as soon as possible.

Don't forget to write, telephone, or telegraph your family and friends outside the area to let them know that the emergency is over and that you are safe. If you fail to let them know, they may waste considerable time and money trying to find you. Let them know where you are and that you are all right.

NEIGHBORHOOD

Possible Problems

My residence is located in:

Megalopolis . . . . ☐ _____

Metropolis . . . . ☐ _____

Major city . . . . ☐ _____

Town . . . . ☐ _____

Country . . . . ☐ _____

Major apartment complex . . ☐ _____

High-rise apartment . . . . . ☐ _____

Condo complex . . . . . . ☐ _____

There are:

Gas utilities . . . . ☐ _____

Sewer lines . . . . ☐ _____

Within five miles of my residence there are:

Railroads/railroad yards . . . ☐ _____

Freeways/turnpikes . . . . . ☐ _____

Main highways . . . . ☐ _____

Seaport . . . . ☐ _____

Riverport . . . . ☐ _____

Airport . . . . ☐ _____

Landing pattern for

major airport . . . . ☐ _____

City sewer lines . . . . . . ☐ _____

City gas lines . . . . ☐ _____

Major manufacturing . . . . ☐ _____

Factories . . . . ☐ _____

Industrial area(s) . . . . . ☐ _____

Chemical plants . . . . . . ☐ _____

Missile/arms manufacturing . ☐ _____

Refineries or storage facilities . ☐ _____

Other . . . . ☐ _____

Armed services:

Base . . . . ☐ _____

Storage facilities . . . . . . ☐ _____

Bunkers . . . . ☐ _____

Planes/fuel . . . . ☐ _____

Armories . . . . ☐ _____

Weapons/gas repository . . . ☐ _____

Missile base . . . . ☐ _____

Other . . . . ☐ _____

Dams/reservoirs/levees

Earthen . . . . ☐ _____

Concrete . . . . ☐ _____

EVALUATION

Wash
"Dry" riverbeds . . . . . . ☐ _____
Terrain in surrounding area
includes:
   Desert . . . . ☐ _____
   Mountains . . . . ☐ _____
   Earthquake faults . . . . . ☐ _____
   Flood plain . . . . ☐ _____
   Rivers/creeks/lakes . . . . ☐ _____
   Ocean . . . . ☐ _____
   Other . . . . ☐ _____
Weather problems could include:
   Severe weather pattern: common/occasional
      Spring . . . . ☐ ☐ _____
      Summer . . . . ☐ ☐ _____
      Fall . . . . ☐ ☐ _____
      Winter . . . . ☐ ☐ _____
   Hurricanes . . . . ☐ ☐ _____
   Tornadoes . . . . ☐ ☐ _____
   Tidal waves . . . . ☐ ☐ _____
   Monsoon . . . . ☐ ☐ _____
   Snow . . . . ☐ ☐ _____
   Ice . . . . ☐ ☐ _____
   Rain . . . . ☐ ☐ _____
   Lightning/thunder . . . . ☐ ☐ _____
   Severe thunderstorms . . . ☐ ☐ _____
   Wind . . . . ☐ ☐ _____
   Seasonal brushfires . . . . ☐ ☐ _____
   Wood fires . . . . ☐ ☐ _____
   Floods . . . . ☐ ☐ _____
   Mudslides . . . . ☐ ☐ _____
   Other . . . . ☐ ☐ _____

Possible evacuation centers (name and location):

_____
_____
_____
_____

Phone numbers:
   Local Red Cross _____
   Local emergency services _____
   Police _____
   Paramedics _____

WORKSHEET FOR

Light	On hand	Buy	Use and replace

Heat	On hand	Buy	Use and replace

Shelter	On hand	Buy	Use and replace

Hygiene	On hand	Buy	Use and replace

Sanitation

Equipment

Morale boosters

Communications

72-HOUR EVACUATION KIT

On hand	Buy	Use and replace

First aid	On hand	Buy	Use and replace

On hand	Buy	Use and replace

Personal	On hand	Buy	Use and replace

On hand	Buy	Use and replace

Special needs	On hand	Buy	Use and replace

On hand	Buy	Use and replace

Special needs (continued)	On hand	Buy	Use and replace

FOOD AND EQUIPMENT

Stress foods	Amount needed	On hand	Need to buy	Cost at store #1	Cost at store #2	Cost at store #3

Compressed food bars	Amount needed	On hand	Need to buy	Cost at store #1	Cost at store #2	Cost at store #3

Trail mix	Amount needed	On hand	Need to buy	Cost at store #1	Cost at store #2	Cost at store #3

Dried foods	Amount needed	On hand	Need to buy	Cost at store #1	Cost at store #2	Cost at store #3

For (name)	For (name)	For (name)	For (name)	For (name)	For (name)	Notes

For (name)	For (name)	For (name)	For (name)	For (name)	For (name)	Notes

For (name)	For (name)	For (name)	For (name)	For (name)	For (name)	Notes

For (name)	For (name)	For (name)	For (name)	For (name)	For (name)	Notes

FOOD AND EQUIPMENT

Freeze-dried foods	Amount needed	On hand	Need to buy	Cost at store #1	Cost at store #2	Cost at store #3

Instant meals	Amount needed	On hand	Need to buy	Cost at store #1	Cost at store #2	Cost at store #3

Snack-sized canned goods	Amount needed	On hand	Need to buy	Cost at store #1	Cost at store #2	Cost at store #3

Snack foods	Amount needed	On hand	Need to buy	Cost at store #1	Cost at store #2	Cost at store #3

For (name)	For (name)	For (name)	For (name)	For (name)	For (name)	Notes

For (name)	For (name)	For (name)	For (name)	For (name)	For (name)	Notes

For (name)	For (name)	For (name)	For (name)	For (name)	For (name)	Notes

For (name)	For (name)	For (name)	For (name)	For (name)	For (name)	Notes

FOOD AND EQUIPMENT

Baby foods and formula	Amount needed	On hand	Need to buy	Cost at store #1.	Cost at store #2	Cost at store #3

Special diet	Amount needed	On hand	Need to buy	Cost at store #1	Cost at store #2	Cost at store #3

Drink mixes	Amount needed	On hand	Need to buy	Cost at store #1	Cost at store #2	Cost at store #3

Water and beverages	Amount needed	On hand	Need to buy	Cost at store #1	Cost at store #2	Cost at store #3

For (name)	For (name)	For (name)	For (name)	For (name)	For (name)	Notes

For (name)	For (name)	For (name)	For (name)	For (name)	For (name)	Notes

For (name)	For (name)	For (name)	For (name)	For (name)	For (name)	Notes

For (name)	For (name)	For (name)	For (name)	For (name)	For (name)	Notes

FOOD AND EQUIPMENT

Small containers	Amount needed	On hand	Need to buy	Cost at store #1	Cost at store #2	Cost at store #3

Water containers	Amount needed	On hand	Need to buy	Cost at store #1	Cost at store #2	Cost at store #3

Utensils	Amount needed	On hand	Need to buy	Cost at store #1	Cost at store #2	Cost at store #3

Equipment	Amount needed	On hand	Need to buy	Cost at store #1	Cost at store #2	Cost at store #3

TO BE PURCHASED

For (name)	For (name)	For (name)	For (name)	For (name)	For (name)	Notes

For (name)	For (name)	For (name)	For (name)	For (name)	For (name)	Notes

For (name)	For (name)	For (name)	For (name)	For (name)	For (name)	Notes

For (name)	For (name)	For (name)	For (name)	For (name)	For (name)	Notes

CARE-IN-A-CRISIS PLAN

Condition	What I do	What cooperating family does for me	What I do for cooperating family
A spouse isn't home			
Parents aren't home			
Children aren't home			
You or your neighbor is a widow, widower, handicapped person, single parent, or elderly person, or has specific needs			
You have a large family			
You live alone			
A family member must be left behind			
Other			

Discuss the following subjects and list your decisions about each one.

Specific assignments during an evacuation _____

_____

Specific assignments at a shelter _____

_____

The need to stay in the shelter rather than wandering off _____

_____

How to find the Missing Persons area of the shelter _____

_____

Whom to let know and how to let someone know you have been separated from your family _____

_____

_____

Who might be able to help you at the shelter _____

_____

_____

How to recognize badges, uniforms, and people in authority _____

_____

_____

Which neighbors to seek out for help_____

_____

_____

How to use the buddy system (make assignments) _____

_____

_____

How and when to use the evacuation kit _____

_____

_____

Ways to help others at the shelter _____

_____

_____

What to look for and listen for (announcements, all clear, etc.) _____

_____

_____

Remember to take the evacuation kits of all household members with you to the evacuation center! Those away from home should be directed to the shelter area.

How to Help Those Not Involved with Care-in-a-Crisis

Offer reassurance, security, comfort.

Take stranded children to the evacuation shelter with you. Immediately report to those in charge the names and ages of those you have brought. Keep the children with you until parents or older brother or sister (whom you know) claim them.

Take an older person with you to the shelter. Immediately report to those in charge. Keep the person with you until a family member is located.

Look after a widow, widower, or handicapped person who might be living alone near you.

Help provide transportation to a shelter.

Let others know who is with you so that their family members will find out.

Help another family with children.

Help another family with an invalid or elderly person.

Be aware of children (and adults) struggling with fear or insecurity. You can offer reassurance, calm, and comfort.

Seek out those in charge and offer assistance where it is needed.

FAMILY INFORMATION

Description of Family Members

Date filled out _____

Name	Birth date	Height	Coloring	Hair color	Eye color	Special needs

Schedule of Family Members

	Name	Address	Phone	Time
Work				
Work				
Babysitter				
Daycare				
School				
School				
School				
School				

Your family's emergency meeting place (away from home):

_____

Person, family, or families assigned as cooperating family to look out for your family in your absence:

Name _____

Address _____ Phone _____

Relative (or close friend) to be informed about which cooperating family is assigned to look out for your family during a crisis:

Name _____

Address _____ Phone _____

Person(s) or families you and your family are assigned to look out for as a cooperating family:

Name _____

Address _____ Phone _____

Name _____

Address _____ Phone _____